M000234396

HOMOEOPATHY
IN VETERINARY
PRACTICE

K. J. Biddis, MRCVS

HOMOEOPATHY IN VETERINARY PRACTICE

Enlarged Second Edition including:

A Practical Guide to Prescribing

The Treatment of Goats
(by G. Macleod, MRCVS, DVSM)

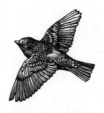

THE C. W. DANIEL COMPANY LIMITED
1 Church Path, Saffron Walden
Essex, England

First published in Great Britain in 1987
© K. J. Biddis 1987

© *The Treatment of Goats*
G. Macleod 1980

ISBN 0 85207 196 5

Reprinted 1995

Printed in the United Kingdom

Set in Souvenir by MS Typesetting,
Castle Camps, Cambridge and printed by
Hillman Printers (Frome) Ltd, Frome, Somerset

Contents

PREFACE

The call for a second edition of this work is very gratifying to me.

The chapter *Practical Guide to Prescribing* has been added as a result of suggestions made by veterinary colleagues and others, who have been using homoeopathic remedies without having available any written information on prescribing and its attendant ramifications.

With the use of this book all animals, both large and small, can be treated, because the majority of ailments can occur in species of any size. The enlarged Therapeutic Index now also covers some conditions that are peculiar to large animals, e.g. actinomycosis, foot-rot, laminitis, mastitis etc.

I am indebted to Mr G. Macleod, MRCVS, DVSM for permission to include his excellent chapter on *The Treatment of Goats*.

A PRACTICAL GUIDE

There is no mystique associated with homoeopathic prescribing. It is not a programme of therapy based on the emotional or spiritual levels. It is basically a difference in treatment and not in diagnosis. Homoeopathy is the giving of a very small dose of a substance, possibly a poison, which in a large dose would cause symptoms similar to the illness presented for treatment. Hence the Greek origin of the word Homoeopathy, which means 'Like the Disease'. In order to find a homoeopathic substance, or remedy as it is termed, whose symptoms match up as closely as possible to the symptoms of the illness, it is necessary to ascertain not only in great detail how that particular animal is manifesting the text-book symptoms but also any concomitant symptoms which in themselves would not be regarded as diagnostic. For example, one dog with gastroenteritis may keep craving for just a few laps of cold water which are vomited about five minutes later; it is also very restless. Another dog with the same ailment may keep craving for long draughts of cold water at long intervals and not vomiting for some time later and unlike the other dog, is resting for long periods, only rising to either drink or vomit. They are exhibiting their thirst, due to dehydration, in different ways and neither these nor their other concomitant symptoms of restlessness or long periods of rest are diagnostic symptoms of gastroenteritis. It is only with such details that one can begin to build up a sufficiently comprehensive 'symptom' picture with which to align with a similar 'remedy' picture. Homoeopathic treatment can be prescribed in three different ways:-

Firstly, acute (including per-acute) prescribing, where the symptoms always bear a very close similarity and only have very slight individual variation, for example in per-acute pyrexia or severe physical trauma.

Secondly, symptomatic or pathological prescribing which is based on the symptoms caused by the lesion.

Thirdly, constitutional prescribing, where the object is to treat the whole animal, which is the method most closely associated with Hahnemann's philosophy and principles. It involves building up a complete picture of the character and constitution of the animal which, in the absence of subjective symptoms, can never be as complete as in human prescribing where the mental, or mind, symptoms are so helpful. Because of the time required to both conduct a full examination of the animal and build up such a picture, this method can only be applied to special appointments, whereas methods one and two can be applied in everyday general practice.

In order to obtain optimum results, homoeopathic remedies, like conventional medicaments, must be given in the correct dosage, frequency and for the correct duration — but there the comparison ends. There is no strength to a homoeopathic remedy but what is known as a potency. Strength of a conventional medicament is indicated by the amount of active ingredient it contains and which is usually varied according to the weight of the animal. Potency can be likened to the voltage required to either start or maintain electrical impulses to a mechanism which, irrespective of its size, can only be activated by low or high voltages according to its requirements.

For acute prescribing the high potencies of 30c to 10m, or even higher, are given in fairly rapid succession, often at ten minute intervals, and then discontinued after an hour or so when improvement is registered — but there is no harm in continuing for longer.

For pathological prescribing the 30c potency is regarded as the norm by a large number of prescribers but those that are more discerning have found that the 6c potency is very suitable for ailments affecting the alimentary canal and for the treatment of transudates and exudates. If the 30c potency does not seem effective then the potency recommended in a veterinary materia medica, which has been arrived at by trial and error, should be considered. The 12c potency is not now often used. The length of treatment varies according to the potency that is employed but, as in acute prescribing there is no harm in extending it. When using the 6c potency the procedure would be to give one dose every six hours on the first and second days, one dose every eight hours on the third and fourth days and one dose every twelve hours on the fifth and sixth days. When using the 30c potency, one dose every six to eight hours on the first day and one dose every eight hours on the second day — a total of six or seven doses should be sufficient, bearing in mind that all remedies go on exerting their action for some considerable time after administration has ceased. Although the length of duration of remedies can be found in Dr Gibson Miller's little booklet on the 'Relationship and Duration of Remedies',

13

one has to bear in mind that the duration is shortened when treating acute ailments and often lengthened when treating the chronic ailments constitutionally.

For constitutional prescribing there are two schools who claim satisfactory results. *The purist Hahnemann school*, the very large group of prescribers, would commence treatment by giving three doses only of 30c potency at eight hour intervals and then wait until either the improvement has stopped or, that there are indications that some of the symptoms are beginning to return; three doses of potency 200c are now given in the same way and then wait again as after giving the 30c potency. This procedure is repeated again and again giving successively potencies of 10m, 50m, Cm and even higher, until the symptoms show no sign of returning. If, of course, the symptoms do not return before reaching those very high potencies, then a cure has been effected and there is obviously no need to keep on going higher. At least one month should elapse between each stage before increasing the potency and if this interval between stepping up the potency becomes longer and longer, possibly approximating the stated maximum duration of the remedy in Dr Gibson Miller's booklet, due to improvement being maintained for longer periods, it is a good indication that a cure will be ultimately effected. There are some phenomena associated with this type of constitutional prescribing which should be noted. Firstly, there may be aggravation of the symptoms of the condition being treated. These 'aggravations' are a good sign and indicate that the remedy is correct; they usually occur two or

14

three weeks after giving the remedy and are followed by further improvement of the ailment. Secondly, symptoms may arise which are manifestations of other ailments that have occurred weeks, months or even years previously. These 'old sores' will subside without treatment and like 'aggravations' are a good indication of the correctness of the remedy. Thirdly, symptoms may arise, during the course of treatment, that have never occurred before but are typical of other symptoms of the remedy itself — check in the Materia Medica. These are called 'provings' and if very severe can be immediately eliminated by giving a much higher potency of the same remedy e.g. two or three doses of 10m or Cm. The use of antidotes, as indicated in Dr Gibson Miller's booklet, are not often needed but are indicated when the apparent 'provings' coincide with a remedy that is either 'complementary' or one of the 'remedies that follows well', or even both. The art of distinguishing between 'aggravations', 'old sores' and the recognition of new symptoms that will require another remedy altogether, is delicate and only comes with practise and experience. This constitutional procedure cannot be expedited by not waiting for each potency to run its course; in fact it might even have the opposite desired effect by causing marked aggravation of the old symptoms which may take many weeks or months to eliminate. *The other school of constitutional prescribers* give a long course, lasting four to six weeks, using a very low potency like a 3x three times a day.

Administration of the remedy. The optimum speed of absorption of the remedy is through the mucous membrane of the mouth — not the stomach — and by finely crushing a tablet in a folded card it can be easily tipped into the mouth. Because the quantity is so small it quickly dissolves in the saliva. As in the human subject, it is known that the sub-lingual area gives the quickest absorption rate but it is hardly likely that the veterinary administrator will be that skilful, or lucky enough, to reach that area. It is inconsequential whether one, two or more tablets are given as a single dose because the total potency received by the animal will still be the same as if only one tablet had been given, in the same way as connecting two or more batteries of the same voltage in *parallel* will give the same voltage output as if only one battery is used. However it might be considered advisable to crush two or more tablets together in order to increase the bulk if it is thought that some of the dose might be spilt during administration. Do not give either food or drink for half an hour either side of administration. This rapid absorption through the mucous membrane of the mouth not only ensures quicker effect but also eliminates the risk of the medicament being lost due to vomiting. When prescribing constitutionally the animal's skin should be checked for residual topical medications, particularly those with a sulphur content because, either licking this surface medicament or its absorption through the skin could interfere with the action of the remedy.

NOTE

These general guidelines should provide the prescriber, especially the newcomer, with a basis from which to work. With experience, some prescribers quite rightly, deviate from these general guidelines particularly when undertaking pathological/symptom prescribing for certain species of animal — a commendable practice if improved results are obtained.

Selecting the Remedy. It is necessary to have other books available for reference. *Firstly*, a Materia Medica; Boericke's 'Materia Medica with Repertory' is recommended; this homoeopathic repertory, similar to Hahnemann's Schema, lists remedies in relation to their symptoms whereas in the materia medica the symptoms are listed in relation to the remedies. The Therapeutic Index at the end of this book lists the remedies in relation to named ailments. *Secondly*, as mentioned earlier, Dr Gibson Miller's booklet 'Relationship of Remedies with Duration of Action'.

For Acute remedy selection a similar procedure to making an allopathic choice is adopted. The Therapeutic Index will list suitable remedies. There is no need to be too selective; for example, if a haemostatic is required, it is better to commence with a good general purpose haemostatic like Arnica, than a remedy which is suggested for bleeding from a specific part of the body as when the haemorrhage is probably associated with less acute or traumatic conditions e.g. for blood from the bowels when one might select Hammelis if it is dark in colour, Ipecac if it is light in colour and Merc corr., if the colour is inconsistent. For fulminating conditions, possibly with pyrexia, Acon nap would be the first remedy of choice. Neither Arnica or Aconitum would be given much consideration when treating

17

pathologically or constitutionally except as initial medication.

For Pathological/Symptom remedy selection the animal's symptom picture will need elaboration, particularly the Modalities of the symptoms. Modalities are the modifying influences, aggravating or ameliorating, which are affecting the symptoms. (The Modalities will be detailed later.) Having completed the animal's symptom picture the Therapeutic Index should be consulted to find some suitable remedies, the details of which will be found in the Materia Medica. *Firstly*, read the Modalities of each of these suitable remedies before reading the full text, because if the Modalities of the remedy are dissimilar or even opposite to the Modalities of the animal's symptoms, then that remedy can justifiably be relegated to a low position on the short list; alternatively, those remedies whose Modalities align well should be given first consideration. *Secondly*, read that section of the text which deals with the location of the ailment. Concomitant symptoms may appear in other parts of the text which may help to confirm the selection being made. There are about 1,250 remedies in Boericke but most prescribers have their own pet list of about a dozen remedies which they have memorised, the knowledge of which is so helpful for prescribing at this pathological/symptom level, e.g. Ars. alb., Bryonia, Hypericum, Merc. corr., Merc. sol., Nux. vom., Puls., Rhus. tox., Sil., Sulph. If only the Modalities of these few remedies could be memorised it would be found quite helpful.

For Constitutional remedy selection a full examination of the animal and building up a complete picture of its character and constitution including past medical history, is essential. In order to obtain this complete picture one should follow the materia medica format by successively taking each system in turn — face, ears, nose and so on, eventually reaching the Modalities which are now applied to the normal reactions of the whole animal and not just to the modalities of the ailment symptoms. For example, one would want to know whether the animal is a 'hot' or 'chilly' type. The chilly types are frequently the thin skinned breeds that are attracted to the warmth of the fire or radiator whereas the hot types always prefer to lie on the coolest part of the floor as far as possible from the source of heat. It is well known that before the era of receptionists or electronic hailing systems the homoeopathic physician would take the opportunity of looking into his waiting room each time he personally ushered in each patient in order to observe the 'types' that were still waiting; the chilly type well wrapped up but sitting as close to the radiator as possible; the hot type sitting near the street door with overcoat already removed; the other chilly type still wearing his overcoat but sitting near the fresh air coming in from the fanlight, obviously enjoying the reflected heat from the radiator but not a hot stuffy atmosphere — a preliminary homoeopathic typing of three patients before they had entered his consulting room, effected purely by observation. It must be remembered that the majority of dogs, whether they are hot or chilly types, enjoy a walk irrespective of the weather being hot or cold and so care must be taken in interpreting their reactions to heat and cold. Lastly, one can now turn to the remedy, slotting its symptom picture into the complete constitutional picture, continually cross-indexing with repertory and materia medica. It may be that a final selection is still unclear due either, to lack of definite answers from the owner or, from marked inconsistencies in the modalities; in such cases it would be usual to adopt one of two procedures, either give three doses of Sulphur 200 at eight hour intervals and review the case again fourteen to twenty eight days later, because Sulphur has the propensity of helping to clear the symptom picture of less important details thus making the selection of the remedy much clearer, or, alternatively, give the selected remedy in the 6c potency three times a day for one week and then review the case again fourteen days after completion of this course; improvement would indicate that it is the correct remedy and should respond to successively higher potencies. Improvement during constitutional prescribing may not initially apply to the ailment itself but in the general well-being of the animal. It is not unusual for the owner to observe that the animal is behaving as though the tablets had acted as a general tonic. This corresponds to the human patients' observation that they feel better in themselves although the ailment has not improved. This constitutional improvement indicates that the correct remedy has been selected.

The Modalities

In constitutional prescribing for human patients, consideration of the subjective 'mind' symptoms is considered essential. In the absence of these subjective symptoms being available to the veterinary prescriber the modalities must assume a pre-eminently important place. When homoeopaths generalise about people or animals being certain types they are referring to their dominant modalities e.g. Arsenic types are chilly and restless, Sulphur types are hot and have an irritable nature. The range of modalities in Boericke is so comprehensive that it is unnecessary to repeat them here other than give examples of some of their veterinary applications. There are six groups of modalities:-

(1) **Thermal** These two tables cover those remedies which are commonly used in veterinary practice. If one had a skin complaint which, taking all other factors into consideration, appeared to be a choice between Sulphur or Psorinum, then the thermal modality of the symptoms particularly and those of the animal in general, could be the deciding factor.

CHILLY types

Symptoms aggravated by cold;
ameliorated by warmth

ARS. ALB.	Hug	GELS.	But not
	the	PULS.	stuffy
NUX.VOM.	fire	SEPIA.	atmosphere

BARYT.CARB.		GRAPH.
CAL.CARB.		KALI. SULPH.
CAUL.	Like	NIT. AC.
HEP. SULPH.	to be	RHUS. TOX.
PLUMB.	covered	SPON.
PSOR.		THUJA
SIL.		

HOT types
Symptoms aggravated by warmth; ameliorated by cold

APIS.		GLON.
CANTH.	Resent	OPIUM
PULS.	covering	LACH.
SULPH.		
ARG.NIT.		

(2) **Physical** These relate to the effects of rest, movement, exertion, posture, etc. The correct interpretation of this modality is important; for instance, 'worse for rest' does not necessarily mean 'better for movement' unless definitely so stated. Pulsatilla symptoms can be aggravated or ameliorated when resting or lying down, this is because Pulsatilla types are known to be changeable and so the physical modalities of this remedy are often inconclusive. The physical modalities of Rhus. tox., on the other hand, are outstanding and consistent; the dog affected with the fibrositis-like syndrone, screaming and staggering around after resting but limbering up with movement, is typical; the symptoms returning again after another period of rest.

(3) **Metabolic** which cover the effects on symptoms of eating, drinking, defaecation, sleeping etc. Some conditions are worse after sleep — as distinct from rest. Lachesis is probably the best known remedy for this particular modality. The onset of some conditions, like petit mal in the dog, frequently occurs when passing from sleep to wakefulness. The sudden uncontrollable desire to defaecate immediately after eating or drinking fits well into the modality of Aloe.

(4) **Chronological** It is noteworthy when listening to clients, to hear of aggravation of

their animals' symptoms recurring consistently at certain times of the day, night, month or even the year. Midnight is a well-known aggravation time for Ars. alb. symptoms; acute conditions like vomiting and chronic conditions like the persistent restlessness of the senile dog, are typical of this remedy's midnight aggravation. The dog that has diarrhoea early every morning but is normal for the rest of the day is probably a Sulphur type. It is well known that many mentally disturbed people have an aggravation of their symptoms every twenty eight days, particularly at full moon — hence the word *lunatic*. Silicea symptoms often recur every twenty eight days and it has been used successfully for the cure of the seizures of grand-mal epilepsy in the dog when this modality has fitted. Rhus. tox. should always be considered for the treatment of those skin complaints which recur yearly — not necessarily with the advent of warmer weather.

(5) **Meteorological** The weather would appear to have less influence on animal ailments than it does on human ailments. The increase of heat in the summer months is really a thermal modality and is not appreciated by 'hot' types whose skin disorders are aggravated. There are some dogs that scratch continuously after exercising in the rain and these usually respond well to Rhus. tox.

(6) **Psychological** Here again, of much more importance in human homoeopathy where the subjective symptoms outlined in Boericke under 'mind' can be fully utilised and their modalities carefully noted. Psychosomatic illness in the animal is usually caused by frustration and it is the symptoms

and modalities of the frustration that have to be treated even though the causal factor cannot be eradicated e.g. separation from owner, temporary or permanent.

Nosodes

These are remedies that are made from diseased tissues, or, from associated organisms, or, from bacteria, or, viruses in culture form. They are used mainly in the 30c or 200c potencies. They were originally used therapeutically, Psorinum being a good example, forming a useful addition to the homoeopath's armamentarium. The use of some nosodes prophylactically became popular in the 1920s and were designated as Oral Vaccines, a term which has since been dropped when the dominant conventional school of medicine commenced using their own Oral Vaccines. The use of a nosode as a prophylatic can be compared to the administration of an immune or hyperimmune serum and should be regarded in this light.

MATERIA MEDICA

ALOE

Great urgency to evacuate the contents of the rectum immediately after eating or drinking. Aloe 30 should be given three times a day for four or five days.

ALUMINA

Constipation when the stool is large, whitish and crumbly; the rectum is dry and bleeding through straining. Alumina 30 should be given every four to six hours for at least four or five days.

APIS

For any lesion where, due to the stretching of the skin, the appearance is swollen, red and smooth. The grossly swollen and shiny red eyelids associated with a foreign body in the eye respond readily to this remedy making easier the removal of the foreign body. Sudden violent skin irritations, with or without swelling as in urticaria, on any part of the body. Apis 30 should be given every fifteen minutes until the condition subsides.

ARNICA

Trauma of any type e.g. blows, falls, bruising, shock after road accidents, bite wounds, cerebral haemorrhages, concussion, disc protusion, fractures, grazes, haemorrhage, muscle injuries, traumatic orchitis, traumatic pain, teeth extraction, shock. When given immediately after the trauma, it minimises pain, shock and other sequelae local or general. For haemorrhage, Arnica Cm, or lower if this is not available, should be given every ten minutes until five doses have been given. Arnica 30 given half an hour before surgical interference and if possible, every eight hours on the previous day, ensures minimal bleeding and shock, followed by rapid, uneventful and painless recovery. Quite obviously Arnica will not repair a fracture but if given as soon as possible it aborts the associated soft tissue swelling by checking the haemorrhage and bruising, reduces the pain and shock, thereby facilitating immobilisation. It has been used for shock that had caused a budgerigar to stop talking.

ARSENICUM ALBUM

Marked restlessness is the great feature of this remedy. It has always been regarded as the horse's remedy, particularly the nervous animal, constantly moving about, very restless and prone to take fright. The old Arsenic habit of the Styrian mountaineers arose from the discovery of its power of strengthening the muscles, the respiratory system and the disgestive system — all desirable features that would be desired by a horsekeeper particularly if the horse had a 'staring coat'. Three doses of Arsenic 30 are indicated for such an animal. Repetitive craving for just a few laps of cold water which are vomited a few minutes later can be assuaged with Arsenic 30 given every two hours until four or five doses have been given. (With Merc., vomiting — Corr. or Sol. — the desire is for long draughts of cold water which are not immediately vomited; also the animal is not restless). In addition to the dry staring coat, scurf can be treated with Arsenic 30 once a day for a week but if there is exfoliation of very large scurfy flakes

Ars. iod. 30 given in the same way may prove more effective. The senile dog which persists in walking around the house all night, occasionally barking to be let outside for no apparent reason and only resting for about five minutes at a time will respond to three doses of Arsenic 30.

For coryza, in cats, particularly those who are 'chilly' types, Ars 3 given four times a day has been used with considerable success in the treatment of the coryza associated with the respiratory type of 'cat flu'.

BACILLINUM

This nosode has been used successfully in the treatment of ringworm in cattle by giving Bacillinum 200, two doses, with an interval of one month between each dose. Animals that are 'poor doers' for no accountable reason can benefit from Bacillinum 30 one dose daily for one week.

BELLADONNA

Whereas the incidence of heat-stroke from the direct rays of the sun is very low in animals at least one has in Belladonna a remedy which is clearly indicated. In the early stages of a severe case, Bell 30 should be given every ten minutes until the twitchings and convulsive movements subside. If this is followed by a severe apoplectic state characterised by a change to constricted pupils and heavy stertorous breathing then Op. 30 should be given in the same way. For heat-stroke from hot air, as from a closed car see Glonoine.

29

BORAX

Sensitivity to sudden or loud noises like fireworks or thunder. Animals so affected will shiver, try to hide, sometimes bark incessantly and try to escape from the owner if outdoors. Dogs in Australia have been observed in this state of fear for some hours before the occurrence of an electric storm. Treatment is more effective when given prophylactically; it is obviously not possible to anticipate a thunderstorm, but a week's course of Borax 3x, three times a day every four weeks during the summer months would help those dogs that are terrified of thunderstorms. The fright caused by road vehicles with inadequate silencers can be offset by giving this remedy. Whereas Gels. and Arg. nit are the established human remedies for impending fear and fright, Borax 3x has been found a useful prophylactic before the animal visits either the veterinary surgeon's or the stripping operator's premises for which some animals harbour an inherent dislike; three doses should be given the day before and one dose on the morning of attendance. Borax 3x is the best potency.

BRYONIA

To normalise lactation when the milk flow is poor due to over-engorged breasts, one dose of Bry. 3c should be given every two hours. When engorgement is due to weaning, Bry 3c should be given every six hours.

Aggravation of symptoms by movement, however slight, is the dominant modality of this remedy. Rheumatism, particularly muscular, which is worse with exercise and better with rest, should be given Bry 30 three times a day for two days. A dry cough which is aggravated by even the slightest movement such as changing position when half asleep should be given Bry 30 three times a day for three or four days.

CACTUS

The constrictive pain associated with Angina Pectoris causing the animal to scream and fall over, a condition more likely to occur in the older dog, can be effectively treated with Cact. 30 giving three doses at eight hour intervals. Treatment may need to be repeated every two or three months.

CANTHARIS

This is the outstanding remedy for acute cystitis and other urinary upsets. For chronic cystitis use Sarsaparilla. Burns, including sunburn, and scolds respond well. Canth can be used in all potencies 6c – 10m and as frequently as the acuteness of the condition dictates.

CAPSICUM

This remedy suits the dog which is normally ill-disposed towards strangers and which is now fretting through being parted from its owner. This separation may be purely temporary whilst the owner is away on holiday. Give two doses of Caps 10m with a twelve hour interval between each dose or 3 doses of 30c if the higher potency is not available. If it appears ineffective try Acon., Ign., or Staph. in the same way.

CARBO. VEG.

The formation of excessive quantities of gas in any part of the digestive tract calls for the use of this remedy. Older dogs that persistently pass offensive flatus when resting should be given Carb. v. 6 three times a day for four days. Carb. v. are 'chilly' types and so if the animal is a 'hot' type Sulph should be given for this condition. The rapid formation of gas in the stomach occasionally met in the larger breeds such as the Great Dane should be given Carb. v. 6 every ten minutes until the condition subsides. Colchicum is an alternate remedy for this condition.

CAULOPHYLUM

The action of this remedy on the female generative organs is outstanding and can be used both prophylactically and therapeutically. When given prophylactically it normalises parturition; bitches should be given one dose of Caul 30 once a week for three weeks before whelping and cattle should be given Caul 30 once a month for three months before calving. Its special sphere during labour is (1) when the contractions do not come regularly; (2) when the contractions cease from exhaustion and (3) when the contractions are obviously abnormally painful; Caul 30 should be given every fifteen minutes for each of these three abnormalities. Pyometra responds well to Caul 30 given three times a day for six days or longer.

CAUSTICUM

Caust. 30 given three times a day for six days is excellent for urinary incontinence caused by excitement or coughing, or arising during first sleep as in puppies. Dogs suffering from Bell's Palsy should be given

Caust 30 once a day for six days, to be repeated two weeks later if necessary. Treatment of chorea in the dog is indicated when the condition has become static and if there is a co-existing partial paralysis then Caust. 30 once a day for ten days is particularly indicated; do not repeat for at least three weeks. Thuja is usually the remedy of choice for warts but Caust will often clear those warts that are resistant to Thuja.

CHELIDONIUM

Essentially a remedy for the treatment of symptoms associated with liver dysfunction or liver disease. Dogs which are prone to sub-acute liver upsets which commence with thirstlessness, inappetance and frequent yawning — a typical symptom of liver upset, which is much more apparent than the yawning associated with the Nux v. liver upsets. These symptoms may continue for four or five days before the onset of vomiting. The vomit is yellow or yellow/green in colour. Chel. 30 should be given four times a day for four or five days. Irrespective of the cause, jaundiced patients will benefit from this remedy given four times a day as with the other liver upsets.

CICUTA VIROSA

For spasmodic nervous affections. Of particular use in fits and convulsions of undetermined origin in puppies and young dogs. Cic. v. 30 should be given every eight hours until six doses have been given.

COCCULUS

This remedy given either on its own or combined with Tabacum overcomes the various distressing symptoms of travel sickness. It is particularly indicated when vomiting and excitement are prominent symptoms, whereas Tabacum is indicated when there is quietness, quivering and depression with little or no vomiting. Cocculus on its own is usually quite sufficient. Give Cocc. 12 or 30 three times on the day prior to travel and once before setting out.

COLCHICUM

Ailments benefiting from this remedy are usually both acute and severe. It is indicated when there is rapid accumulation of gas in the stomach in small animals and in the rumen of cattle (bloat). Colch. 6 should be given every fifteen minutes for six doses.

CONIUM

Effective in one of the symptoms of old age, namely, loss of strength and stiffness in the hind legs. This condition is seen most frequently in the larger breeds, particularly the Alsatian. The history is typical; the condition has been slow and insidious in onset; in the early stages the dog experiences difficulty in rising off the hind legs from the sitting or lying position, particularly after a long rest; there is a tendency for the legs to tremble, more noticeably at the end of the day. After a few months the owner finds it helpful to assist the dog to its feet. On examination the dog is normal apart from partial atrophy of the hind leg muscles caused by inactivity. Con. 6 should be given three times a day for ten days and repeated every four to six months when necessary.

CROTON TIGLIUM

Painful wet eczematous conditions that occur around the scrotum or in the external ear; the irritation is intense and scratching is very painful; the animal resents the gentlest touch or application to the affected part. Crot. t. 30 should be given three or four times a day.

EUPHRASIA

This remedy has a wide application in disorders of the eye. Its effectiveness in chronic inflammatory conditions such as keratitis is outstanding. Used topically on its own or as an adjunct to internal medication, it can be used for catarrhal conjunctivitis, coryza, corneal ulcers and corneal opacities. Internally Euph. 6 every two hours; externally, dilute 10 drops of the tincture in 30 ml of water and use four times a day.

GELSEMIUM

Emotional excitement leading to bodily ailments is the leading veterinary indication. Its action centres upon the nervous system. The emotional tension or excitement that the male dog undergoes when it is under the same roof without access to a bitch that is 'in season' leads to a deterioration of both its mental and physical condition. The dog is obviously ill through worrying. Gels. 3 should be given three times a day for one week.

GLONOINE

For heat-stroke due to hot air rather than direct rays of the sun, of the type seen in animals that have been shut in a closed vehicle. Should also be used in animals that have collapsed after over-exerting themselves on a hot sultry day. Glon. 30 or higher every ten minutes. As with Belladonna, it should be followed with Opium if the animal becomes comatose.

GRAPHITES

Of particular use is the treatment of chronic wet eczema occurring in the bends of the limbs, groins and behind the ears especially in lethargic, obese and middle-aged dogs. Also for seborrhoea (grease) in horses. Graph. 30 should be given three times a day for one week. A black diarrhoea in dogs, not accompanied by any other sign of ill-health nor with an imbalance in the diet should be given Graph 30 three times a day for six days.

HEPAR SULPH

For acute and sub-acute conditions associated with pus formation (use Silicea for chronic sepsis). Suppuration is hastened by the low potency and aborted by the high. In the former give Hep. 2x every four hours; in the latter five Hep. 200 every six hours. Pus in the anterior chamber of the eye (hypopyon) even if inspissated, can be dispersed with Hep. 30 given three times a day for one week. For sebaceous glands or cysts give Hep. 30 daily for seven days or Hep. 200 twice a day for four days.

HYPERICUM

The great remedy for injuries to nerves, particularly nerve endings. Pinched or crushed toes: injured dew claws and other nail injuries which are all extremely painful, obtain rapid relief from Hyper. 30 four times a day. The prolonged sensitivity in an amputated digit could be given similar treatment. The very painful lacerated wound, which can be even more painful than the puncture wound of Ledum, is relieved with Hyper. 30 every six hours.

IGNATIA

The animal that pines because it is separated from its owner has always been a problem. All the material kindness that is bestowed upon it has no apparent effect and it maintains its state of melancholic brooding. Two doses of Ign. 10m should be given with a twelve interval between each dose; 30c or 200c can be used if 10m not available.

IPECACUANHA

For the control of retching and vomiting associated with 'fur balls' in cats Ipecac. 6 should be given half an hour before each meal.

IRIS VERSICOLOR

An excellent remedy for the symptoms associated with affections of the pancreas, particularly the diarrhoea. Iris v. 6x should be given three times a day for at least three or four weeks.

LAUROCERASUS

Very useful for the control of the irritating 'cardiac cough' that affects many old dogs. Laur. 6x should be given three times a day, reducing to twice a day as the condition responds.

LEDUM

Essentially for painful puncture wounds. The pain from a puncture wound is often out of all proportion to the size of the lesion, as a person who has been bitten by a cat will confirm. One would use Ledum in preference to Arnica when there is no laceration or surface bruising but infinitely more pain. Ledum, like Arnica, inhibits pus formation. Led. 30 should be given every six hours until six doses have been given.

MERC CORR

The quantity of this remedy that is used in canine practice probably exceeds that of all other remedies; this is probably due to the fact that disorders of the digestive tract, particularly the bowels, are encountered more frequently than other ailments. Other than in surface conditions, the intense thirst for large quanities of cold water gives a strong pointer for the use of this remedy. This water is vomited some time later, often after the dog has been resting: (note the marked contrast from Ars Alb. The colour of the vomit or diarrhoea varies between yellow and green and sometimes streaked with blood. There is a marked tenesmus following evacuation. Merc. c. quite supersedes the use of any other therapy for the treatment of tenesmus. Merc. c. should be given every six hours for the first two days and the frequency decreased over the next few days. Per-acute haemorrhagic gastro-enteritis should be given Merc c. 200 every fifteen minutes until the symptoms show marked signs of subsiding before reducing the frequency, the course of treatment lasting for four or five days. Merc. c. 6 can be given with other compatible remedies when there is marked tenesmus associated with strangury or prostatic enlargement

MERC. SOL

Although this remedy can be used for the same conditions as Merc. c., it is not so effective when the symptoms are severe; it should certainly be used if Merc. c., is not immediately available. Excessive lachrymation or salivation; coryza with or without sneezing; simple or ulcerative stomatitis should be given Merc. s. 6 every four to six hours. Inflammation of the kidneys, particularly chronic interstitial nephritis, can be helped with Merc. s. 6 four times a day for seven days followed by Merc. s. 30 once a day for a further seven days. Chronic eczemas in older dogs associated with sub-clinical nephritis should be given Merc. s. 6 three times a day for ten days. For acute wet eczema occurring during the summer months Merc. s. 200 should be given every six hours until ten doses have been given and then reduce the frequency; this procedure obviates completely the necessity to clip, clean or use topical applications. (Petroleum for similar eczema in the winter months).

NAT MUR

Indicated in the treatment of a certain transient type of change in disposition that is peculiar to both cats and dogs. The normally placid animal is apparently enjoying being stroked and fondled when it suddenly bites the owner viciously; the incident is only transient and is usually followed by a period of sulking. Nat. m. 30 three doses only will usually eradicate this pecularity for some months. There is little evidence that the veterinary use of this remedy is as extensive as it is in human medicine where some physicians regard it as the constitutional remedy *par excellence*.

NITRIC ACID

Sneezing, with or without epistaxis, often occurs without any obvious cause. Nit. ac. 30 should be given every ten minutes. For coryza, particularly if it is blood stained when it is associated with sinusitis should be given Nit. ac. 6 three times a day for at least six to eight days. The post-distemper/ paradistemper thickening of the skin of the nose and the pads should be given three doses of Nit. ac. 30 once a month.

NUX VOMICA

For simple and uncomplicated vomiting when the vomit is clear or white and there is absence of thirst, Nux. v. 6 should be given four times a day for five or six days. When there is constipation with frequent urging and straining Nux v. 30 should be given three or four times a day; Nux. v. is contra-indicated if there is absence of straining. Persistent hiccough can be treated with Nux. v. 3 given every ten minutes. The onset of painful disc disorder associated with taut muscles and varying degrees of paraly-sis should be given Nux. v. 30 every two hours until relief is obtained. Animals that are frightened by loud traffic noise can

sometimes be helped by giving Nux v. 30
twice a day for four days.

OPIUM

When an animal is comatose due to apo-
plexy, concussion or heat-stroke Op. 30
should be given every ten minutes. The
memory of severe fright, which may have
occurred some years previously, can be
helped with Op. 30 twice a day for three
days.

PHOSPHORIC ACID

There is a condition that occurs in puppies
and kittens that responds quickly to this
remedy. It is characterised by an almost
clear, watery motion that is passed involun-
tarily, soiling the bed and running down its
legs when it moves; the animal is otherwise
in good health. Phos. ac. 6x should be
given three times a day for five days even
although the condition may appear relieved
after the first twenty four hours. The stud
animal that has been over-used and is
suffering from deficient sexual power should
be given Phos. ac. 6x three times a day for
ten days.

PHOSPHORUS

Liver dysfunction in the young energetic
animal (differentiate from hyperthyroidism)
which is losing weight and apparently passing a larger volume of normal faeces then
food consumed should be given Phos. 30
three times a day for two days. Repeat the
treatment every four weeks if the weight
gain is not maintained. Post-operative shock
and/or haemorrhage can be counteracted

by giving Phos. 30 every t.fteen minutes. Like Borax and Nux. vom, it has been helpful in alleviating disturbances of the nervous sytem caused by loud noises.

PHYTOLACCA

A glandular remedy of particular use for the veterinary treatment of the mammary gland. For mastitis in diary cows Phyt. 30 should be given three times a day for four days and then twice a day for the next two days. Quiescent nodules in the canine and feline mammary gland can be treated by noting the chronological modality of this remedy, Phyt. 200 should be given once every twenty eight days on three occasions, then 10m in the same way — a six month course of treatment that is worth trying.

PLUMBUM

For the treatment of chronic interstitial nephritis in old animals, particularly in cats. Commence by giving Plumb. 6 three times a day for one week; this can be followed by Plumb. 30 once a day for one week.

PODOPHYLLUM

For the treatment of diarrhoea which is always accompanied with considerable flatus. Due to the flatus the motion has to be passed with such urgency that the dog is unable to reach its usual place for defaecation. The defaecation is noisy, due to the flatus, but there is no tenesmus nor does the dog appear distressed. The motion is brown, bubbly and very watery. Give Pod. 6 or 30 three times a day for five days.

PULSATILLA

This remedy has a variety of useful applications particularly for the female genital organs. For amenorrhoea Puls. 30 should be given three times a day for one week. For the bitch with irregular menses the same procedure should be adopted by commencing four months exactly after the commencement of the previous 'season'. The bitch that is a typical Puls. type constitutionally may, at confinement, benefit equally as well with this remedy as Caulophyllum, giving Puls. 30 every half an hour during labour. Phantom pregnancy can be treated with Puls. 30 given three times a day for one week. Enlarged prostate, Puls. 30 three times a day for seven days; repeat three weeks later. Merc. cor 6 can be given at the same time if there is marked tenesmus. Subacute middle ear infections should be given Puls. 200 morning and evening for three days and repeated after an interval of fourteen days. The dog that always dislikes being left alone is a typical Puls. type. The degree to which the dog demands the company of the owner determines when an inordinate affection has developed into a neurosis. The dog that barks incessantly until the owner's return, much to the neighbours' annoyance is a typical example; four doses of Puls. 200 should be given at twelve hour intervals and repeated after an interval of one month if necessary. In many ailments Sepia can be used as an alternative treatment for the female generative organs where the temperament of the patient is more applicable, bearing in mind that Puls.

patients are constitutionally affectionate types whereas Sepia types are the opposite.

RUTA

For the treatment of harder tissues such as sprained joint ligaments and bruised bones when, following initial Arnica medication, Rut. 30 should be given every eight hours for two or three days. For chronic sprains see Strontium.

RHUS TOXICONENDRUM

The patient that responds well to this remedy suffers from the type of rheumatism that is always worse after rest — particularly after a long rest such as a night's sleep. Although relatively young, about three or four years of age, it has difficulty in moving off its bed and eventually staggers around like an old man but limbers up with movement. The discomfort on beginning to move may evince a whimper or even a scream. Sometimes the back is arched due to involvement of the abdominal muscles and the dog is reluctant to defaecate because, assuming the required position causes pain in these muscles. The neck muscles are also sometimes affected. Rhus. tox. 30 should be given three times a day for four days. The dog that is suffering from the ill-effects of an infrequent bath — general stiffness and malaise — should receive a similar course of treatment. Selected skin conditions that recur yearly should be given Rhus. tox. 200 three times a day for three or four days.

SABINA

As this remedy has a special action on the uterus it is of considerable use in the treatment of sub-acute or chronic endometritis, Sabin. 12 should be given three times a day for ten days.

SILICEA

This remedy is indicated in chronic or sub-acute sepsis (for acute sepsis see Hepar. Sulph.). Where the lesion is exuding a thin blood stained fluid, Sil. 6 should be given three times a day for six days. This remedy can be very slow acting and at least two weeks should elapse before repeating the treatment. Very resistant cases will respond to increasingly higher potencies. Schirrous cord and similar exuberant granulations are comparatively rare nowadays but respond to Sil. 30 three times a day for four days. Adhesions should be given Sil. 6 three times a day for eight days. Foreign bodies, particularly the smaller type which are encountered in the eye or foot are extruded by this remedy. Its use to effect the extrusion of 'spear grass' from feet considerably reduces the necessity for surgical interference, Sil. 30 should be given three times a day for four to six days. Interdigital cysts, chronic sepsis in open jonts and bones and anal gland disorders should be given Sil. 6 three times a day for one week and after an interval of two or three weeks given increasingly higher potencies with suitable intervals between each. Painless swollen glands and cysts should be given Sil. 30 three times a day for four days before repeating, if necessary, with a higher potency three weeks later. Symptoms caused by pathological changes in joint or bone tissue can often be completely eliminated in such conditions as Perthes's disease, hip dysplasia and navicular disease. The modalities of Sil. are very similar to those of the Dachshund e.g. the desire to be completely covered, and so Sil. should always be thought of when treating this breed. Epilepsy grand mal has been treated with success — the twenty eighth day modality; three doses of Sil. 30 should be given at eight hour intervals, giving at least a four to six weeks interval before repetition of the same potency.

SPONGIA

The dry, chronic and sympathetic cough of organic heart disease can be relieved with this remedy giving Spon. 6 three times a day for at least eight days. It is a difficult condition to control and Naja tripudians and Lauroceausus might be considered if Spon. appears ineffective. Some pet dogs when put into boarding kennels develop a persistent cough due either to persistent barking or acquiring an endemic throat infection; Spon. 6 given three times a day has often proved effective. Coccus cacti is a useful alternative remedy for this irritating type of cough.

STRAMONIUM

For the cat that has developed the unpleasant habit of 'wetting' around the house Stram. 30 should be given once a day for seven days.

STRONTIUM

For chronic sprains, particularly chronic sprained tendons of the horse and greyhound which cause recurrent symptoms even after prolonged rest periods Stront. 30 should be given daily for seven days. Potencies up to M of 10m can be given after appropriate intervals between each course.

SULPHUR

The majority of long-haired dogs do not enjoy either natural or artificial heat and skin disorders of this type of dog are nearly always aggravated by heat. Dry, non-parasitic hyperaemic skin disorders will benefit from a short course of this remedy, irrespective of what subsequent treatment is prescribed giving Sulp. 200 daily for seven days. The dog that persistently passes an evil smelling flatus when sleeping in the evenings in a warm room should be given Sulph. 6 twice a day for seven days. Pyrexia and hyperpyrexia associated with viraemias respond to this remedy, often with no subsequent secondary infections or other sequelae — an advantage over Aconitum — by giving Sulph. 200 every six hours for the first four days and then every eight hours for the next three days.

SYMPHYTUM

The routine use of this remedy after a fracture has been immobilised ensures that the non-union factor is entirely eliminated. In addition, optimum healing of the fracture is effected with the result that racing animals are able to resume training in a much shorter time; Symph. 6 should be given three times a day for the first ten days after immobilisation. Traumatic injuries to the eye that have been caused by an obtuse body and where there is bruising and pain, are quickly relieved with this remedy by giving Symph. 6 four times a day for two or three days.

THIOSINAMINUM

An excellent remedy for dissolving scar tissue. Adhesions following major extensive internal surgery are a prominent indication and stricture of the rectum/anal ring have yielded to this remedy. Thiosin. 6 should be given three times a day for ten days and repeated again after an interval of three weeks.

THUJA

All types of warts, from buccal papillomata in the young dog, to multiple, widespread, irritating and bleeding verucca in the old dog, can be treated with this remedy. Thuj. 200 should be given twice a day for four days and repeated three weeks later if necessary. Some dogs suffer long-term ill-effects from vaccination. These ill effects are manifested in the young dog in a variety of ways, such as recurrent non-parasitic skin disorders, lethargy, fickle appetite etc. Thuj. 30 should be given three times a day for two days. The retension cyst that occurs under the tongue — ranula — can be dispersed with this remedy either by giving Thuj. 3 five or six times a day for four days or, Thuj. 200 three times a day for four days.

URTICA URENS

For the regulation of milk secretion. To stimulate milk secretion Urt. ur. 30 one dose only; to suppress secretion Urt. ur. 1x every six hours until relief is obtained.

TREATMENT OF GOATS
BY HOMOEOPATHY
by George Macleod, MRVCS, DVSM

ALIMENTARY AND DIGESTIVE SYSTEMS

The more important conditions we should consider are conditions affecting the mouth, the rumen and the intestines with, in addition, peritonitis and affections of the liver.

A. **STOMATITIS:** Inflammation of the mucous membrane of the mouth includes extension to the gums and tongue and is characterised by redness; salivation and possibly ulceration. Prominent among remedies used to control this condition are MERC. SOL., BORAX and ACID NIT. The mercury salts produce a picture of salivation with or without ulceration. Borax produces aphthous lesions on the tongue papillae with ropy saliva, while nitric acid is associated with small flat ulcers along the gums and around the lips. For treatment Merc. Sol. or Merc. Cor. should be used in 6c potency, giving a dose three times daily for five days. Borax should also be used in 6c potency in the same way, while Acid. Nit, is best used in a higher potency — e.g. 200c, giving one dose per day for one week.

B: **INDIGESTION:** This is usually a disturbance of physiological function, no pathological changes taking place. Simple indigestion shows as lack of appetite with a slight increase in the rate of respiration. The faeces may be hard or watery, depending on the nature of the food partaken. Rumenal contractions may be reduced when the dung is dry or increased when diarrhoea is present. Rumenal impaction produces a doughy feeling with reduced stomach movement. The chief remedies to be considered in treatment are as follows:

(1) ABIES CANADENSIS 6c: This is a useful remedy when overeating is the cause. Abdominal flatulence is common. Dose: one every two hours for 4 doses.

(2) NUX VOMICA 12x: Indicated when arising from indigestible fodder. Constiptation is invariably present. Dose: as for Abies.

(3) COLCHICUM 6c: Rumenal tympany is usually present when this remedy is indicated. The origin frequently lies in too much green food. Dose: as for Abies and Nux.

C: **ENTERITIS:** Inflammation of the intestinal tract may follow acute indigestion or be secondary to some septic state, such as mastitis or metritis. Diarrhoea occurs with evidence of pain. The animal refuses food and shreds of mucus may be present in the faeces along with blood. Main remedies required are:

(1) ACONITUM 30c: Should be given early in the condition if possible. It will help allay shock and calm the patient. Dose: one every 20 minutes for 4 doses.

(2) ARSENICUM ALBUM 1M: Restlessness and a worsening of symptoms towards midnight call for this remedy. The stool may have a cadaverous odour. Dose: one very hour for 4 doses.

(3) COLOCYNTHIS 6c: Symptoms of abdominal pain are very pronounced. The animal may arch its back and draw its legs under the abdomen. Dose: one every ½ hour for 4 doses.

(4) MERC. CORR. 200c: Mucous dysenteric stools are present. Symptoms are

worse in the period from sunset to sunrise.
Dose: one x three times daily for 3 days.

D: **PERITONITIS:** This condition is rarely
primary, being usually a sequal to some
condition such as gastritis, mastitis or metritis. Lack of appetite accompanies a rise in
temperature and pulse rate, together with
an increase in respiration. The back
becomes arched and a painful grunt is
present on expiration. The peritoneal covering can be felt as a hard board-like mass on
pressure over the sub-lumbar fossa. Remedies include:

(1) ACONITUM 6c: Will relieve pain and
anxiety if given early. Dose: one every ½
hour for 6 doses.

(2) BELLADONNA 1M: The animal has a
staring look and feels hot. Head shaking
may occur. The pulse is hard and full. Dose:
one every ½ hour for 4 doses.

(3) BRYONIA ALBA 30c: Tenderness over
the abdomen is extreme, but deep pressure
relieves symptoms. Dose: one every three
hours for 4 doses.

(4) CANTHARIS 30c: indicated when
there is severe inflammatory involvement of
the whole peritoneal covering. Blood may
be present in stools. The condition is often
dependent on an underlying cystitis or
nephritis. Dose: one every ½ hour for 6
doses.

(5) RHUS TOX 1M: Relief is evident on
movement. Redness of visible mucous
membranes is a guiding symptom. Dose:
one every two hours for 4 doses.

E: **BLOAT:** Acute tympany of the rumen is
a specific form of indigestion which can arise
suddenly when gas in the rumen is pro-
duced faster than it is eliminated. Lush

pastures in spring or autumn may give rise to it as well as the intake of large amounts of grain. A reduced intake of roughage will contribute to bloat, as the rumen depends on a sufficient quantity for its proper function. Treatment includes the following:

(1) ANTIMONIUM CRUDUM 6c: A useful remedy in frothy bloat, which comes on quickly after eating. Dose: one every hour for 4 doses.

(2) CARBO. VEG. 6c: This is suitable for less acute cases. The animal may show signs of restlessness. Dose: one every hour for 6 doses.

(3) LYCOPODIUM 1M: A useful remedy in chronic or recurrent cases. Probably dependent on malfunction of liver metabolism. Dose one per day for 7 days.

(4) COLCHICUM 200c: Already mentioned.

F: **DIARRHOEA:** Can arise from various causes and there are many remedies available to deal with this, according to symptoms. Slimy diarrhoea containing blood and accompanied by straining indicates MERC. CORR. Thirst for small quantities of water, together with harsh dry coat and restlessness suggests ARSEN. ALB. If the diarrhoea is watery and forcibly expelled, PODOPHYLLUM could be the remedy. CAMPHOR is indicated when the animal is in a state of collapse and body temperature is low, with black stools. VERATRUM ALB. is also associated with collapse, but the stools are greenish. Autumn diarrhoea, which may arise when cool evenings follow a warm day, usually responds to DULCAMARA. In all cases CHINA should be given, together with the appropriate remedy, as it restores strength after loss of body fluids. Other remedies which might be needed include IPEPCAC., CROTON TIG., PYRO-GEN., PHOSPH. ACID, ALOE and RHEUM.

In dealing with intestinal complaints, it may be useful to mention the control of worms by homoeopathic means, although advice on this is not often sought. If it is, the owner is frequently discouraged by the time involved in treatment, the remedies having to be given frequently over a few days; e.g., ABROTANUM 1x (a useful remedy) needs to be administered four times daily for 4 days and repeated again in 3 weeks. Other remedies which are used are CINA MARI-TIMA and CHENOPODIUM. Liver fluke is particularly difficult to deal with and if you wish to try treating it homoeopathically, I would suggest tackling it by concentrating on remedies which have a selected action on the liver; e.g., CHELIDONIUM, PHOS-PHORUS and BERBERIS VULGARIS and LYCOPODIUM. The stimulating action of these remedies on the liver tissue and bile ducts may help indirecly in controlling fluke.

Depraved appetite in the goat may require remedies like CALC. PHOSPH., CALC. CARB., PHOSPH., COBALTUM or CUPRUM. Animals which are short of lime will frequently eat bones and here the two Ca. remedies will help. Phosph. is indicated when leathery objects are chewed, while the trace elements of Co. and Cu. are associated with a particular type of pica seen often in marginal land grazings.

RESPIRATORY DISEASES

The only conditions which need con-cern us are congestion of lungs, pneumonia and pleurisy.

A: **CONGESTION OF LUNGS:** This condition may arise from an increased blood-supply when it is termed active, or when there is interference with blood-supply — passive congestion. Exposure to cold weather is a common cause, as also is transportion over long distances. There may be a rapid rise in temperature. Breathing becomes laboured and frothy saliva is evident, accompanied by a grunting sound when breathing out. The severity of the breathing depends on the amount of fluid present. Treatment includes the following:

(1) ACONITUM 6c: For the early feverish state. Dose: one every ½ hour for 4 doses.

(2) AMMONIUM CAUSTICUM 30c: A useful remedy for the control of moist coughing. Dose: one x three times daily for 3 days.

(3) ANTIMONIUM TART. 30c: Indicated if there is pneumonia threatening. The animal usually coughs up mucus. Dose: as above.

(4) ANTIMONIUM ARSENICOSUM 30c: A valuable remedy when the congestion is worse on the left side. The patient prefers to lie down and there may be an accompanying oedema of the brisket. Dose: one x three times daily for 5 days.

(5) AMMONIUM CARB. 30c: More suitable for right-sided congestion, usually venous in origin. Dose: as for the previous remedy.

B: **PNEUMONIA:** This may take various forms but the commonest type is broncho-pneumonia which can arise suddenly or be more insidious in onset. Exposure to cold and damp are predisposing causes, while fatigue and transportation are contributory factors. Infectious agents include viruses and pasteurella and corynebacteria. A rise in temperature accompanies coughing, depression and lack of appetite. Grunting and mouth breathing are present in severe cases. The following remedies should hlep:

(1) ACONITUM 6c: Should always be given early, if possible, when by itself it may abort the disease process. Dose: one every ½ hour for 4 doses.

(2) ANTIMONIUM TART. 30c: For moist coughing with patchy distribution of lung lesions. There is usually abundant mucus. Dose: one x three times daily for 3 days.

(3) BERYLLIUM 30c: A useful remedy when the underlying condition is more severe than symptoms would suggest. Slight movement brings on coughing. Dose: one night and morning for 4 days.

(4) BRYONIA 30c: Indicated when the animal is disinclined to move. Pressure over the chest walls brings relief. Dose: as above.

(5) DROSERA 9c: For those cases when a spasmodic cough is present. Coughing appears to come from the upper respiratory region. Dose: as above.

(6) PHOSPHORUS 200c: When coughing comes from deep down in the chest. There may be rust-coloured sputum. Respirations are quick and shallow. Dose: one every three hours for 4 doses.

The above remedies may also be needed for pleuritic conditions. Pleurisy is seldom seen as a primary condition, as it is usually secondary to pneumonia or pericarditis.

DISEASES OF URINARY SYSTEM

The two conditions which we need look at are *Pyelonephritis* and *Cystitis*. The former is an infection of the kidney which may be brought on by ascending infection from the urinary tract, or be dependent on the septicaemic condition. It may give signs of colic while the urine becomes blood-stained and contains purulent material. Treatment includes the use of one or other of the following remedies:

(1) HEPAR CULPH. 200c: Indicated when there is extreme tenderness over the loins. It is a suitable remedy for acute cases. Dose: one every two hours for 4 doses.

(2) SILICEA 200c: More suitable for a long-standing case. Dose: one x twice weekly for 2 weeks.

(3) MERC. CORR. 30c: Slimy blood-stained urine containing mucus shreds and pus indicates this remedy. The pus is frequently greenish-tinged. Dose: once daily for one week.

CYSTITIS: Inflmmation of the bladder may be primary or secondary — the latter being more common. It may also be acute or chronic. The acute form is usually bacterial in origin, while the chronic form may be associated with gravel or sand in the urine. Frequent urination is the commonest sign, the urine containing blood. There is usually difficulty in passing urine; arching of the back and kicking at the abdomen are seen. The main remedy for treating the acute case is CANTHARIS 30c, indicated when there is severe straining with signs of pain. One dose should be given every hour for 4 doses. The remedy COPAIVA 6c is indicated when there is a large amount of mucus in the urine, which has a sweetish smell. Dose: one every two hours for 4 doses.

For the chronic case, the two most important remedies are THLASPI BURSA 6c and UVA URSI 3x. The former is associated with gravel or sand and is a good remedy for dissolving these deposits, allowing urine to pass freely. Uva Ursi gives a urine which is consistently slimy, associated with pain intermittently. Both these remedies should be given daily for ten days or a fortnight.

AFFECTIONS OF THE SKIN

These include Ringworm and Eczema, and Alopecia. *Ringworm* is a superficial fungus disease and is more common in the younger animal. The lesions usually assume an annular shape and in severe cases may be large and extensive. Itching is considerable and the coat becomes dry and scaly. The remedy which I have found most successful in dealing with ringwork in animals if BACILLINUM 200c. This is a nosode prepared from tuberculous material and should be given in monthly doses for 3 months. Another useful adjunct remedy is TELLURIUM 9c. The ring-shaped lesions suggest that this remedy might give good results, but I have no personal record of it in treating ringworm. SEPIA 200c has also given good results, the dose being the same as for Bacillinum.

ECZEMA: Seen as bare patches, either inflamed and red or as bare white lesions. Sometimes little is seen and the owner's attention is drawn to the animal simply scratching, leading to loss of hair. There are a large number of remedies available for the treatment of eczema, chief among them being SULPHUR, ARSEN. ALB., SELE-

NIUM, HEPAR SULPH., and SULPHUR IODIDE. SULPHUR should be considered when lesions are red and shiny, and should be given in the 200c potency twice per week for 2 weeks. ARSEN. ALB. is indicated when the coat is harsh and dry and lustreless, with considerable itching, giving rise to scaly deposits like dandruff. It is good in all potencies from 6c to 1M.

If secondary infection supervenes in an eczematous lesion, HEPAR SULPH. may be needed particularly so when there is an associated extreme sensitivity of the surrounding area. The 200c potency should be used and repeated twice daily for 5 days. SELENIUM is associated with miliary eruptions which itch, giving rise to flat ulcers with a corresponding loss of hair around the part. The lesions tend to be worse around the joints and 30c potency is indicated, once per day for 2 weeks. SULPHUR IODIDE is a useful follow-on remedy after the use of these others — it will frequently extend the action and brings more lasting results.

These are only a few of the many remedies available, and reference should be made to a standard Materia Medica for information on others; some important ones being: PSORINUM, TELLURIUM, KALI ARSENICUM, NAT. MUR., and RHUS TOX.

AFFECTIONS OF THE FEMALE REPRODUCTIVE TRACT

Space forbids a detailed look at specific diseases which may affect the female goat, and we will confine our remarks to infertility and troubles associated with parturition. Infertility may have its origin in ovarian dysfunction or in abnormalities of the uterus and Fallopian tubes. It may be permanent or temporary.

TEMPERAMENTAL FACTORS: Refusal to mate is uncommon, but when it does, it is worth trying the remedy SEPIA in 200c potency. This remedy has been used successfully in this connection in the mare and bitch, but I have no personal experience of it in the goat. It should be remembered just the same.

ABORTION OF FOETUS AT AN EARLY STAGE: Apart from specific diseases, non-specific abortion may also occur. This may take the form of an early discharge and may require the remedy VIBURNUM OP. 30c, which has a good reputation for treating early miscarriage. Other useful remedies are CAULOPHYLLUM 30c and SEPIA 200c. One dose per week for 3 weeks should be given for these three remedies.

ENDOCRINE DYSFUNCTION: In one or other of its manifestations this is probably the most common breeding irregularity. Examples are: SUB-OESTRUS or SILENT HEAT when the remedies SEPIA 200c, PULSATILLA 30c, PLATINA 30c and ALETRIS FARINOSA 30c, may be needed. SEPIA should be given in all cases — one dose per week for 3 doses. PULSATILLA and PLATINA are both excellent ovarian remedies, the former associated with vaginal discharges, and the latter with reddish sediment in the urine. They should be used as for Sepia. ALETRIS is more a uterine remedy, general atony being present with occasional bleeding, the blood being dark and membranous.

ANOESTRUS: For animals which fail to come into season, the following remedies may prove useful: SEPIA 200c, one dose only. PULSATILLA 30c, one dose per week for 3 weeks. CALCAREA PHOSPHORICA 6c, is frequently associated with vaginal discharges. IODUM 30c is a useful remedy for excessively lean animals with abnormal appetite and poor coats.

CYSTIC OVARIES: If this complaint is suspected, the following remedies may help: APIS MEL 6c, MUREX PURPUREA 30c and NAT. MUR 30c. Thes have all given excellent results in similar conditions in cattle. Dose: once a week for 3 doses.

FAILURE TO HOLD SERVICE: This is usually due to ovulatory failure during an otherwise normal heat. The following remedies will all be found useful: SEPIA — a single dose. PULSATILLA 30c — when there may be an accompanying creamy discharge. OOPHORINUM 6x — this ovarian extract in potency can be used in conjunction with any of the other remedies.

RETAINED PLACENTA: Not often seen in goats, but when it does occur, the remedies SABINA 6c, PYROGENIUM 1M and PULSATILLA 30c are all useful. I have found SABINA the most useful and it should be given four times in 24 hours. PYROGEN may be needed if the animal shows systemic symptoms of illness accompanying retention.

METRITIS: Inflammation of the womb may arise after parturition (puerperal fever), resulting in severe illness. There is an initial rise in temperature followed by lack of appetite. Respirations are increased and the animal remains recumbent. The pulse may be weak and thready or full and tense. Discharges are not always present, but if they are, they usually contain dark blood. The following remedies will be found useful:

(1) ACONITUM 6c: Should be given at once and repeated every ½ hour for 6 doses.

(2) BELLADONNA 1M: Indicated when the pulse is full and bounding, the pupils are dilated and the animal feels hot all over. The dose is the same as for Aconite and these two remedies can safely be alternated if need be.

(3) ECHINACEA 3x: When systemic involvement is rapid and signs of septicaemia are present. Temperature remains high and respirations are rapid and shallow.

(4) PYROGEN 1M: The guiding signs for the remedy are high temperature alternating with or accompanying a weak thready pulse. Putrid discharges are usually present, together with a cold body surface.

(5) SABINA 6c: When dark blood-stained discharges are present. This remedy acts best when the metritis follows from retained placenta.

(6) LACHESIS 30c: If the condition manifests itself in a haemorrhagic form with a bluish discolouration of visible parts, this remedy will prove effective. There may be an accompanying swelling of the throat region.

MASTITIS: While dealing with post-partum troubles we can look at the problem of udder inflammation. The causes of mastitis are varied and we need not conern ourselves with details of these. Acute, sub-acute and chronic forms of mastitis are met with — general signs in all cases, including changes in milk secretion, leading to clots and abnormalities of udder shape, etc.

The acute form frequently accompanies parturition and also in less severe form, when the animal is going dry. Swelling of the udder may take the form of a slight oedema or be seen as a hot painful enlargement of the gland.

The chronic form shows fibrous inclination of the gland in the region of the milk cistern, and the milk itself shows small clots.

All outbreaks of mastitis call for the employment of various remedies, according to difference in symptoms, and the animal's reactions. Among the commonest remedies employed are the following cases:

ACUTE CASES:
(1) BELLADONNA 1M; Indicated post-partum when the gland is hot and painful, and there are accompanying systemic symptoms of full pulse and hot skin. One dose should be given every hour for 4 doses.

(2) ACONITE 6x: This can profitably be combined with the preceding remedy, and alternated with it in the same dosage.

(3) APIS MEL 30c: A useful remedy for those cases showing an excess of oedema in the gland and surrounding areas. Dose: one every two hours for 4 doses.

(4) BRYONIA 30c: Indicated when the udder tissue is hard and indurated. Chronic forms showing fibrosis may need this remedy. Dose: in acute cases, one x three hourly for 4 doses. In the chronic form, one

x twice weekly for 4 weeks.

(5) PHYTOLACCA 30c: A very good remedy for all forms of mastitis, as it has a special action on glands in general. Acute and chronic cases may need one dose x three times daily for 2 days, followed by one dose every second day for 3 doses.

Other remedies for mastitis which are occasionally used are CALC. FLUOR 30c, AURUM and BELLIS PER. The last two being useful if damage has occurred from bruising or a blow. HEPAR SULPH. also for septic mastitis. A useful remedy for stimulating milk secretion after parturition is URTICA URENS 6x, one dose x three times daily for 3 or 4 days.

If blood appears in the milk, remedies IPECAC 30c and PHOSPHORUS 200c should be remembered — a daily dose of either, usually giving good results — of the two, IPECAC is the most commonly employed.

MINERAL DEFICIENCIES

Trace element deficiency can take different forms, but if the feed is adequate and grazing good, this should not present too many hazards. Calcium deficiency is a special case and this may show after kidding, when the mother remains recumbent and may need Ca. injections. To supplement this homoeopathically and to prevent central nervous system involvement, CALC. PHOSPH. 30c should be given at the same time. This remedy, if given during the last third of pregnancy, will help prevent such deficiencies arising — one dose per week being sufficient.

MISCELLANEOUS CONDITIONS

HEAT STROKE: This may occur if goats are subject to intense heat and have no access to shelter. It can affect the brain and cause delirium. A useful remedy to combat this is GLONOINE 30c, giving one dose every hour for 4 dozes. BELLADONNA 1M may also be needed if brain symptoms such as delirium occur; the dosage being the same.

KETOSIS: An acetonaemia-like condition may arise in heavy yielding goats after parturition, when appetite becomes lost and most foods are rejected. Dung becomes hard and slimy and there may be a bitter taste from the milk. The chief remedy in treatment is LYCOPODIUM 1M which has a direct action on the liver which is at the root of the trouble.

FOOT ROT: As you are aware, goats like hard dry ground, and if subjected to grazing in muddy or infected land, may contract foot-rot, as sheep do. Apart from paring away infected horn, the remedies SILICEA and NAT. MUR. may be needed. SILICEA 30c is probably the most widely used remedy for this — a dose per day for one week, helping to harden the hoof. A foot-rot nosode exists for prevention.

WARTS: These take various forms, from small sessile warts which appear sometimes on the udder and teats of young animals to pedunculated jagged-looking warts which may appear in clusters. The former type usually yield to CALC. CARB. 30c, and the latter to THUJA 6c. THUJA Ø is useful also for painting over and around these angle-berry warts.

INFECTIOUS KERATITIS OR CONTAGIOUS OPHTHALMIA: This is caused by a specific germ and is analogous to the condition in cattle (New Forest Disease). Early symptoms include running eyes with a slight opacity of the cornea. At this stage the remedy KALI HYDRIODICUM 200c will be of use. If the condition is allowed to develop to the stage of severe opacity, SILICEA is probably the most useful remedy — one dose of 200c potency being given twice weekly for one month. Secondary infection leading to purulent ophthalmia may need ARGENT. NIT 30c, MERC. SOL. 200c or HEPAR. SULPH. 200c. In all cases affected eyes should be bathed once or twice daily with a 1/10 dilution of Calendula.

NAVEL ILL, LEADING TO JOINT ILL: Although I have not encountered this trouble among goats, I presume it may occur if kids are born in unhygienic surroundings. The umbilical cord should be dipped in iodine if this condition is considered to be a hazard, and the remedy STREPTOCOCCUS 30c used. This is a nosode and should be given daily for 5 consecutive days.

REARING OF YOUNG KIDS: All young animals should be given a course of CAL. PHOSPH. 30c when they are growing and developing. This remedy is more useful than any other for ensuring good bone development and guarding against deficiency diseases, such as rickets and other bone abnormalities. CALC. FLUOR. 30c is also useful in this respect, its use in helping to harden bone and reducing the likelihood of fractures. These remedies should be given twice weekly for the first 3 months after weaning.

CARE OF THE FEMALE DURING PREGNANCY: Apart from the normal management and good food there are certain remedies which can be used to guard against different hazards, and ensure a safe and trouble-free confinement. The remedy VIBURNUM OP. 30c will be of use in those animals which have previously shown miscarriage early in pregnancy. One dose should be given per week for 4 weeks after service. The two main remedies to ensure easy parturition are CAULOPHYLLUM 30c and ARNICA 30c. Each should be given once per month and an extra dose given during the last week. BELLIS PER. 200c is a good remedy for prevention and treatment of bruising if parturition is difficult.

SPRING FEVER: This is not really a feverish condition, but a scurvy-like condition of the skin and coat which becomes greasy and shows scaly flakes at times. Remedies which could prove useful are THUJA 6c — one dose per day for 14 days, suitable for greasy skins; and ARSEN. ALB. 1M — once per day for one week; more suitable for dry scaly skins.

FALSE PREGNANCY (sometimes called Cloudburst): This can be a troublesome condition and can last quite a long time. If a goat has shown this particular problem in the past, an attempt should be made to prevent it recurring, and the remedy SEPIA 200c will prove useful — one dose per week for 3 weeks being given. This should be followed by the remedy PULSATILLA 30c — once per day for one week. Together, these two remedies will meet most ordinary cases, but other remedies, such as PLATINA, PALLADIUM and CAULOPHYLLUM may be needed. Treatment as such, once the condition is established, will be determined by the particular symptoms displayed, but SEPIA and the nosode OOPHORINUM will cover the majority of cases seen.

GOAT POX: Pox viruses affect animals in different degrees and virulence, and fortunately this trouble is mild in the goat. The pox syndrome shows as a series of lesions starting with papules and going on through vesicular, pustular and scab formation before healing. The lesions affect the teat and udder and are best treated with the remedy ANT. CRUD. 6c in the early papular stage along with the nosode VARIOLINUM 30c. The latter should be given once per day for 3 days, and the former night and morning for one week. The later pustular stages are more effectively treated with THUJA 6c — once per day for 10 days. In contrast, goats can be protected by VARIOLINUM 30c — one dose per day for 3 days or so.

PREGNANCY TOXAEMIA: As in sheep, this troublesome condition is very difficult to treat. Fortunately it is by no means as common in the goat as in the ewe. It is a condition which should, if possible, be prevented by feeding the goat a liberal amount of good quality hay, together with concentrates in the last six weeks of pregnancy. For actual treatment, the remedy PHOSPHORUS 200c will probably be as useful as any, having a direct action on the liver, producing in its provings, a fatty degeneration of liver tissue analogous to that which occurs in pregnancy toxaemia. This should be given daily for 10 days.

ORF OR CONTAGIOUS ECTHYMA: This is a virus disease which produces scab-like lesions around the mouth of young animals and also in the teats, udders and inner thighs of older animals. The preliminary feverish symptoms are seldom seen and it is first noticed by the appearance of the scabs. One of the main remedies used in treatment is ACID NIT. 200c — one dose per day for one week will help clear most cases in the young animal. A different remedy will probably be needed for lesions on the teat and udder and thighs, and I think the most useful one here is RHUS TOX 1M, a daily dose for one week. An Orf nosode could profitably be combined with these remedies, giving one per day for 3 days.

COCCIDIOSIS: This is a specific infection which produces intestinal lesions leading to dysentery, and the appearance in the faeces of whole blood. It is usually confined to the young animal and can cause losses if not properly treated. The main homoeopathic remedies I have found useful in treatment are IPECAC., MERC. CORR. and the bowel nosode SYCOTIC CO. I would suggest SYCOTIC CO 6c, one dose per day for 3 days, combined with IPECAC. 30c one x twice daily for one week. If the stool remains mucoid and thin after treatment,

MERC. CORR. 200c will probably be needed — one dose per day for 5 days.

POISONOUS PLANTS: The plants which have proved to be most toxic are Ragwort, Clematis, Laburnum, Laurel, Rhododendron, Yew, Box and Privet. Treatment of any poisoning is very much a matter of being guided by symptoms displayed, and as these may change rapidly, a variety of remedies may be needed. Once successful case treated for Rhododendron poisoning involved the two remedies NUX. VOM. 1M and RHUS TOX. 6c. I think it would be good practice to give all cases of poisoning a short course of NUX VOM. 1M, one dose every hour for 4 doses. This will cover most digestive symptoms in the early stages. Other remedies which could be indicated are COLCHICUM, COLOCYNTHIS and PODOPHYLLUM. Ragwort has a specific action on the liver and remedies such as CARDUUS MARIANUS and LYCOPODIUM could be indicated. Treatment of poisoning requires a good working knowledge of the Materia Medica and reference should be made to it, taking all objective signs into account. I admit this is not an easy problem for the layman.

In discussing plant (or other poisoning) I would point out that treatment by the potentised plant, e.g. Rhododendron in Rhododendron poisoning is not always indicated. The provings of any remedy may be quite different to the poisonous symptoms of that substance. For instance, I was asked why I did not use Rhododendron in potency when treating the goat which was poisoned by that plant. The answer is that the symptoms the goat displayed were not that of Rhododendron in provings. One must always remember that Homoeopathy depends for successful treatment in prescribing a remedy most similar in its provings to the disease in question.

THERAPEUTIC INDEX

ACETONAEMIA
Cic.; Lyc.; Nux v.

ACTINOBACILLOSIS & ACTINOMYCOSIS
Asaf.; Hekla; Kali iod.; Nit.ac.

ADHESIONS
Sil.; Thiosin.

ANAEMIA
Ars.; Calc.phos.; Carb.v.; China; Cina.; Cob.; Ferr.; Kali c.; Nat.m.; Plumb.ac.; Sil.; Sulph.

ANAL GLANDS
Bellis; Dulc.; Ecchin.; Hep.; Pyr.; Sil.

ANASARCA & ASCITES
Apis; Apocy.; Ars.; Ars.i.; Carb.v.; China; Dig.; Ferr.; Kali c.; Nat.m.; Plumb.ac.; Tereb.

ANGINA
Cact.

ANOREXIA
Lyc.; Nat.m.; Nux v.; Sul.

APOPLEXY
Acon.; Arn.; Bell.; Glon.; Op.; Verat.

ALOPECIA
Alumen; Ars.; Fluor.ac.; Kali ars.; Lyc.; Nat.m.; Phos.ac.; Pix l.; Sel.; Thallium; Ustil.

ARTHRITIS
Apis; Arn.; Bell.; Bry.; Colch.; Led.;
Puls.; Rhod.; Rhus.t.; Ruta.

ASTHMA
Ars.; Baryt.c.; Bell.; Brom.; Carb.v.;
Cina; Cupr.; Grind.; Ipec.; Spig.;
Stroph.; Verat.

BALANITIS
Hep.sulph.; Merc.sol.; Sil.

BILIOUS TENDENCY
Chel.; Nux.vom.

BLOAT
Antim.crud.; Apis.mel.; Carbo.veg.;
Colch.

BRONCHITIS
Acon.; Antim.tart.; Bell.; Bry.; Dulc.;
Ipec.; Lyc.; Mer.sol.; Nat.s.; Puls.; Sticta;
Sul.; Sul.iod.; Spong.; Stroph.

BRUISING
Arn.; Sul.ac.

BURNS AND SCALDS
Canth.; Caust.; Hep.sulph.; Urt.

BUMBLE FOOT
Cal.fluor.

CALCULI
Urinary:- Berb.; Cal.carb.; Cal.phos.;
Canth.; Chimaph.umb.; Lyc.; Oxal.ac.;
Sars.; Solid.
Hepatic:- Berb.; Bry.; Card.m.; Chel.;
China; Lach.; Lyc.

CAPPED HOCK
Arn.; Led.; Rhus.t.

CATARACT
Cann.ind.; Cal.c.; Caust.; Con.; Led.;
Naph.; Phos.; Sec.

CATARRH
Ars.; Merc.c.; Merc.s.

CEREBRAL CONGESTION
Acon.; Apis.; Bell.; Gels.; Glon.; Op.;
Verat.v.

CHALAZION
Staph.

CHOREA
Act.rac.; Agar.; Ars.; Cupr.acet.;
Cal.phos.; Caust.; Ign.; Stram.

COLIC
Acon.; Aesc.; Bell.; Cham.; Cina.;
Colch.; Coloc.; Cupr.; Op.; Plumb.; Sul.

CONCUSSION AND COMA
Acon.; Arn.; Bell.; Glon.; Op.; Verat.v.

CONFINEMENT
Caul.; Puls.

CONSTIPATION
Alumuna; Bry.; Graph.; Lyc.; Nux.v.;
Op.; Plumb.; Puls.

**CORNS & INTERDIGITAL
HYPERPLASIA**
Calc.fluor.; Nat.m.; Sil.

COUGH
Bry.; Laur.; Naja.; Nux.v.; Spong.

Kennel cough Bry.; Coccus.; Spong.

CYSTITIS
Benz.ac.; Berb.; Cann.sat.; Canth.;
Equis.; Lyc.; Nit.ac.; Pareir.b.; Sars.;
Sep.; Staph.; Tereb.

CYSTS
Hep.; Sil.

DEMODEX
Calc.s.; Mez.; Psor.; Selen.; Sul.;
Sul.iod.; Tarent.cub.

DIABETES MELLITUS
Lyc.; Syz.; Sul.

DIARRHOEA & DYSENTERY
Aeth.c.; Aloe; Ars.; Calc.c.; Calc.phos.;
Canth.; Carb.v.; Cham.; Chel.; Cina.;
Colch.; Crot.t.; Cupr.; Graph.; Ipecac.;
Merc.c.; Merc.s.; Nat.s.; Phos.; Phos.ac.;
Pod.; Sec.; Senna; Verat.

DISC DISORDERS
Ars.; Nux.v.; Sil.

EAR DISORDERS
External:- Ars.; Hep.; Merc.s.; Petr.;
Psor.; Sul.; Tell.
Middle:- Merc.s.; Puls.

ECLAMPSIA
Cupr.; Oenanth.

ECZEMA
Ars.; Canth.; Crot.t.; Dulc.; Graph.;
Merc.s.; Mez.; Petr.; Psor.; Rhus.t.; Sel.;
Thuj.; Viol.t.

ENTROPION
Arg.m.; Bor.; Euph..; Merc.s.

EPILEPSY
Aeth.c.; Cic.v.; Cina.; Cupr.; Meli.;
Oenanth.; Phos.; Sil.

EPISTAXIS
Arn.; Bell.; China.; Ipec.; Meli.; Mill.;
Nit.ac.; Sul.

EYE DISORDERS
Bruising:- Symph.
Corneal ulcer:- Euph.; Merc.c.
Corneal ulcer scar:- Kali. bich.
Keratitis:- Arn.; Apis.; Ars.; Ecchin.;
Euph.; Ipec.; Merc.c.; Naphthal.

FISSURES
Graph.; Hep.; Nit.ac.; Petr.; Psor.; Sul.

FISTULAE
Soft tissue:- Hep.; Sil.
Hard tissue:- Hekla; Sil.; Symph.

FITS
Cic.c.; Sil.

FLATULENCE
Carbo.v.; China; Lyc.; Nux.v.

FOOT ROT
Calc.fluor.; Calend.; Hep.; Nat.m.; Sil.

FOREIGN BODY REJECTION
Sil.

FRACTURES
Arn.; Calc.c.; Phos.; Symph.

FRETTING
Caps.; Ign.

GANGRENE
Ars.; Bap.; Carb.ac.; Ecchin.; Lach.;
Pyr.; Sec.

GASTRITIS
Ant.c.; Ars.; Calc.c.; Camph.; Carb.v.;
China.; Colch.; Crotal.h.; Merc.c.;
Merc.s.; Nux.v.; Nat.s.; Phos.; Sul.;
Verat.a.

GLANDS
Anal, Lymph, Sebacious:- Hep.; Sil.

GRAZES
Arn.; Calend.

HAEMATOMA & CONTUSION
Arn.; Bellis.; Chin.s.; Ham.; Ipec.; Phos.

HAEMATURIA
Canth.; Lach.; Tereb.

HAEMORRHAGE
Arn.; Crotal.h.; Ham.;Ipec.; Merc.c.;
Mill.; Nit.ac.; Phos.

HALITOSIS
Arn.; Aur.; Gunp.; Merc.s.; Nit.ac.; Petr.;
Pyr.

HEART DISORDERS
Cough:- Laur.; Naja.; Nux.v.; Spong.
Dilatation:- Arn.; Rhus.t.
Endocarditis:- Ars.; Aur.; Cact.; Conv.;
Naja.
Hypertrophy:- Cact.; Kalm.; Viscum.
Insufficiency:- Apocy.; Arn.; Ars.; Bry.;
Crataeg.; Dig.; Rhus.t.; Stroph.; Verat.

Myocarditis:- Ars.; Aurum; Crataeg.; Iod.
Pericarditis:- Apis.; Bry.; Calc.fluor.

HEAT STROKE
Bell.; Glon.; Op.

HEPATITIS
Card.m.; Chel.; Lyc.

HERNIA
Calc.c.; Nux.v.

HICCOUGH
Nux.v.

INSOMNIA
Ars.; Nux.v.

INOCULATION
Ill effects:- Sil.; Thuj.

JAUNDICE
Bry.; Card.m.; Cean.; Chel.; Chionanth.;
Cholest.; Crotal.h.; Dig.; Lept.; Phos.;
Ricin.com.

LACTATION DISORDERS
Bry.; Urt.ur.

LAMINITIS
Acon.; Bell.; Calc.fluor.; Nux.v.

LARYNGITIS & TRACHEITIS
Ars.; Merc.s.; Spong.

MASTITIS
Apis.; Bell.; Bry.; Phyt.

MENINGITIS
Acon.; Apis.; Ars.; Bell.; Caust.; Circ.v.;
Con.; Gels.; Helleb.; Op.; Verat.v.; Zinc.

MENSES IRREGULARITY
Puls.; Sep.

METRITIS
Arn.; Bapt.; Caul.; Ecchin.; Helon.;
Hydras.; Pyr.; Sabin.; Sep.

NEOPLASMS
Ars.; Baryt.c.; Calc.fluor.; Con.; Sars.;
Phyt.; Thuj.

NEPHRITIS
Acute:- Acon.; Bellis.; Colch.; Phos.;
Sqill.; Tereb.
Chronic:- Aesc.hip.; Aloe; Apocy.; Berb.;
Dig.; Lyc.; Merc.s.; Plumb.; Stroph.

NERVE INJURY
Arn.; Coff.; Hyper.; Ledum.; Ruta.

NERVOUS SYSTEM
Disorders associated with:-
Excitement:- Gels.; Nux.v.
Frustration:- Gels.
Loneliness:- Puls.
Noise:- Bor.; Nux.v.; Phos.
Pain:- Arn.; Hyper.; Ledum.
Phantom pregnancy:- Puls.; Sep.
Pining:- Caps.; Ign.
Senility:- Con.
Shock:- Arn.; Op.; Phos.

ORCHITIS
Arn.; Aur.; Clem.; Puls.; Rhod.; Spong.

OSTEO-MYELITIS
Bell.; Calc.phos.; Hep.; Sil.

PANCREATITIS
Iris.v.

PARALYSIS
Acon.; Caust.; Con.; Gels.; Nux.v.; Op.

PARASITES
Internal:- Cina.; Cupr.; Fil.mas.; Sabad.;
Spig.; Teucr.
External:- Sul.

PERIOSTITIS
Merc.; Mez.; Phos.ac.; Ruta.

PHANTOM PREGNANCY
Croc.; Cycl.; Nux.m.; Puls.; Sep.; Sil.

PLACENTAL RETENTION
Puls.; Sabina.

POLYPUS
Calc.c.; Sang.; Thuja.

PROLAPSE
Rectal:- Cal.c.; Ign.; Merc.c.; Pod.; Sep.
Uterine/Vaginal:- Arg.met.; Lil.t.

PROSTATITIS
Merc.c.; Pareir.b.; Puls.; Sabal.serr.

PURPURA
Arn.; Ars.; Ham.; Lach.; Phos.; Tereb.

PYREXIA
Acon.; Sul.

RANULA
Calc.c.; Fluor.ac.; Thuja.

RHEUMATISM
Articular:- Apis.; Bell.; Bry.; Calc.c.;
Lyc.; Puls.; Rhus.t.; Sul.
Muscular:- Arn.; Berb.; Chel.; Lyc.;
Nat.m.; Rhus.t.; Sep.

SCURF
Ars.; Sul.

SEASON IRREGULARITIES
Puls.; Sep.

SEQUESTRUM
Sil.

SPLEEN DISORDERS
Ceanoth.; Chionanth.

SPRAINS
Arn.; Nat.c.; Rhus.t.; Ruta.; Stront.

STINGS & BITES
Bees & Wasps:- Canth.
Snakes:- Lach.

STOMATITIS
Gunp.; Merc.

STRANGURY
Canth.; Merc.c.; Sars.

SYNOVITIS
Bell.; Bry.; Colch.; Rhus.t.; Sul.

TENESMUS
Canth.; Lil.t.; Merc.c.

TYMPANITES
Abies.canad.; Carbo.v.; Colch.; Graph.;
Nux.v.

URTICARIA
Ant.c.; Apis.; Ars.; Puls.; Urt.ur.

VACCINATION-ILL EFFECTS
Sil.; Thuja.

VOMITING
Ars.; Bry.; Chel.; Ipec.; Merc.; Nux.v.;
Puls.

WOUNDS
Arn.; Calend.; Hyper.; Led.